Lung Cancer Recipe Book

Delicious Life Altering Recipes to Combat Lung Cancer

BY

Daniel Humphreys

Copyright 2019 Daniel Humphreys

License Notes

No part of this Book can be reproduced in any form or by any means including print, electronic, scanning or photocopying unless prior permission is granted by the author.

All ideas, suggestions and guidelines mentioned here are written for informative purposes. While the author has taken every possible step to ensure accuracy, all readers are advised to follow information at their own risk. The author cannot be held responsible for personal and/or commercial damages in case of misinterpreting and misunderstanding any part of this Book

Table of Contents

Introduction 6

    Dairy-Free Blueberry Muesli 8

    Low Glycemic Raspberry Muffins 10

    Oat and Buckwheat Muesli with Pears and Grapes 12

    Arugula, Avocado Tomato Salad 15

    Carrot and Avocado Salad 17

    Beet, Carrot Ginger Salad 19

    Broccoli Salad with Apples and Cranberries 21

    Tomato, Cucumber Red Onion Salad 23

    ACE Salad 25

    Apple Onion Soup 27

    Tangy Tomato Basil Soup 29

    Grandma's Chicken Soup 32

    Beet and Carrot Soup 34

Broccoli and Barley Soup 37

Scandinavian Blueberry Soup 40

Green Tea Mango Blast 42

Catechin-Rich Ice Tea 44

Raspberry Blueberry Smoothie 46

Blueberry Pecan Antioxidant Muffins 48

Low-Fat Apple and Raspberry Crumble 51

Buckwheat Crepes with Prune Compote 54

Flourless Chocolate Cake 57

Rice Pudding with Blueberry Sauce 60

Barley Soup with Beans and Basil 64

Nourishing Nettle Soup 67

Cold Minty Watercress Soup 70

Whole-wheat Pasta with Nettle Pesto 72

Shrimp and Mushroom Risotto 74

Original Bircher Muesli 77

Oat and Wheat Germ Muesli with Apples 79

Conclusion 81

Author's Afterthoughts 82

About the Author 83

Introduction

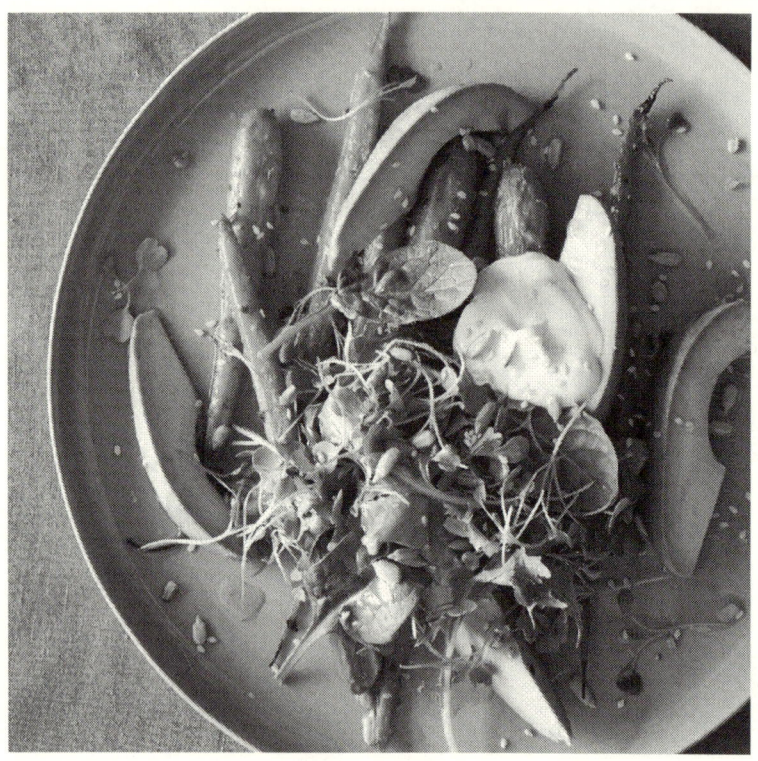

Have you been undergoing treatment for lung cancer, and find yourself having difficulties keeping your food down? The ugly truth is that many lung cancer patients find it difficult to keep their food down due to the pesky symptoms associated with cancer medication, but when this happens, it is important that you keep on trying to eat healthy, food that is easy to digest. Maintaining proper nutrition is a vital part of the cancer recovery process, so consuming nutritional foods will quickly become your go to move. These foods include, but are not limited to:

- Broccoli
- Cod, and other seafood
- Collard greens, and
- Orange juice, to name a few.

Foods like these will assist you in ensuring that your body receives the necessary minerals, and nutrients it needs to prevent or combat lung cancer. Spinning these into delicious recipes will help kick your body back into gear, and provide you with the energy need to push you through each day. There is no time like the present, and at this very moment your present objective is to kick lung cancer to the curb, and these 30 delicious recipes will help you achieve that. So, let's get started.

Dairy-Free Blueberry Muesli

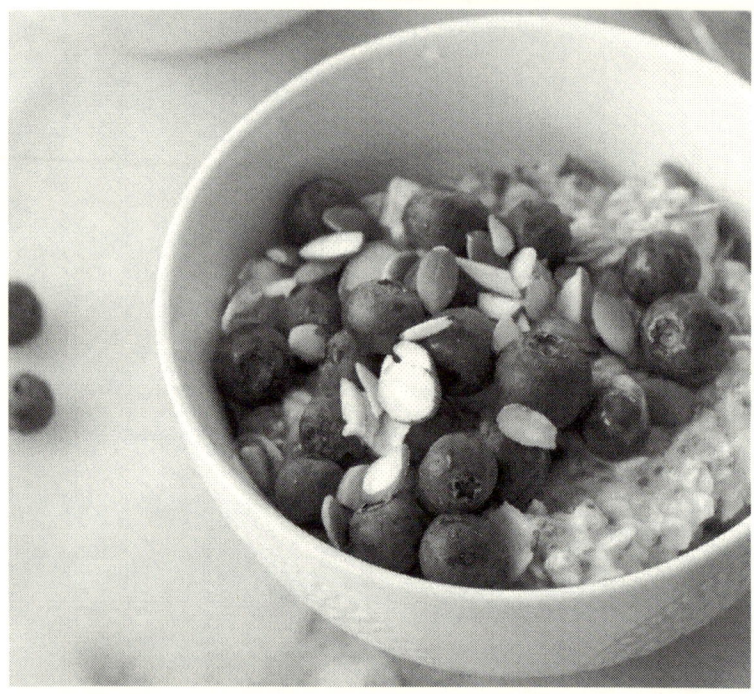

Enjoy this delicious Muesli with a refreshing glass of apple juice to start your morning off right, and get the most of the blueberries antioxidant properties.

Serving Size: 4

Overall Time: 15 Minutes

Ingredients:

- Oats (1½ cups, rolled)
- Walnuts (½ cup, chopped)
- Apples (½ cup, chopped, dried)
- Cinnamon (2 tsp. ground)
- Blueberries (2 cups)
- Brown sugar (3 tbsp.)
- Apple juice (1 cup, to serve)

Directions:

1. Set your oven to preheat to 325 degrees F.

2. In a medium bowl, combine your cinnamon, sugar, and oats. Stir, and transfer the mixture to a lined baking tray, then spread evenly.

3. Set to toast in your oven until lightly golden brown (about 10 minutes, occasionally stirring).

4. Allow to cool slightly, then transfer to a large bowl. Add apples and walnuts. Stir well to fully incorporate.

5. Top with blueberries, and serve with a chilled glass of apple juice.

Low Glycemic Raspberry Muffins

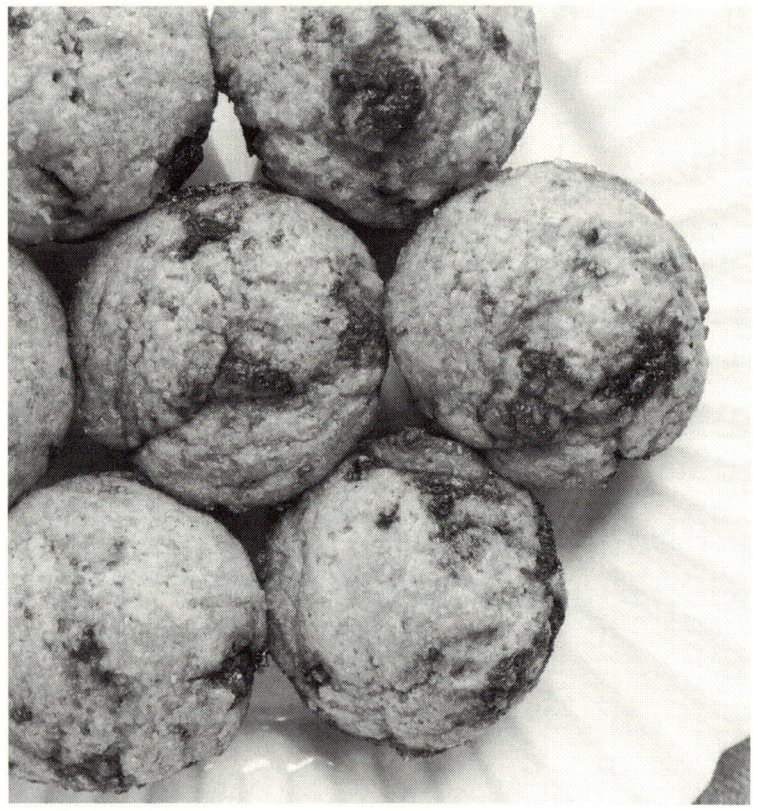

If you love muffins, then there's no need to stop loving them now. Here is a tweaked muffin recipe that with a low glycemic rating that you can try.

Serving Size: 10

Overall Time: 15 Minutes

Ingredients:

- Flour (1½ cups, whole wheat)
- Soy flour (½ cup)
- Baking powder (2 tsp.)
- Brown sugar (1/3 cup)
- Cinnamon (2 tsp.)
- Eggs (2, whites only)
- Soy milk (1 cup)
- Canola oil (2 tbsp.)
- Raspberries (1 cup)

Directions:

1. Set your oven to preheat to 375 degrees F.

2. Add all your dry ingredients to a large bowl. In a separate bowl, add all your wet ingredients, and whisk to combine.

3. Slowly combine both bowls into one, then whisk just until it forms a smooth batter. Add raspberries, and fold.

4. Transfer your batter evenly into a lined muffin tin, and set to bake for about 20 minutes or until done. Enjoy!

Oat and Buckwheat Muesli with Pears and Grapes

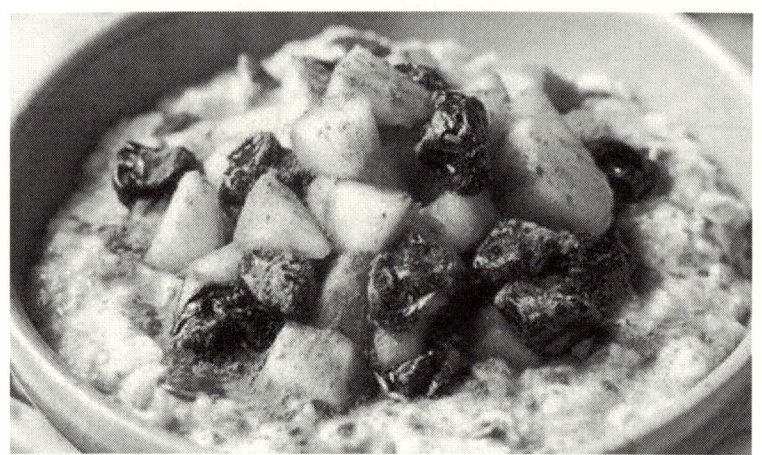

Consuming soaked oats makes it easier for our enzymes to neutralize, and break down the phytic acid it contains so that our bodies can easily absorb its minerals. That is exactly what we do in this delicious Muesli.

Serving Size: 4

Overall Time: 15 Minutes + Soaking time

Ingredients:

- Oats (1½ cups, rolled)
- Buckwheat (1/2 cup, puffed)
- Apples (½ cup, chopped, dried)
- Cinnamon (2 tsp., ground)
- Pears (1 cup, organic, diced)
- Grapes (1 cup, red, halved)
- Brown sugar (3 tbsp.)
- Rice milk (1 cup, to serve)

Directions:

1. Set your oven to preheat to 325 degrees F.

2. Pour your oats evenly onto a lined baking tray, and set to toast in the oven, stirring occasionally until lightly golden brown (about 10 minutes).

3. Allow to cool slightly then transfer to a large bowl. Add water and stir to incorporate. Set in your refrigerator to soak overnight.

4. When ready to eat, remove from refrigerator, add in your remaining ingredients, except rice milk, and stir to combine.

5. Serve with a chilled glass of rice milk.

Arugula, Avocado Tomato Salad

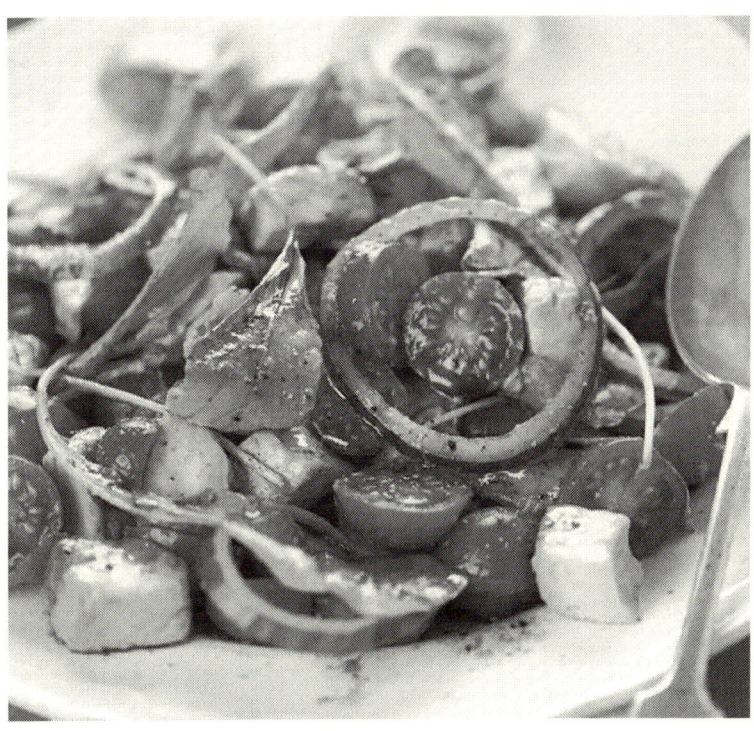

This salad is easy to whip up, low in calories, and delicious while providing just enough phytochemicals to keep your body going.

Serving Size: 4

Overall Time: 10 Minutes

Ingredients:

- Arugula (3 cups, baby, rinsed)
- Cherry tomatoes (2 cups, halved)
- Sun dried tomatoes (1/4 cup, chopped)
- Olive oil (2 tbsp., extra virgin)
- Balsamic vinegar (1 tbsp.)
- Avocados (2 small, pitted, sliced)
- Salt, and pepper (¼ tsp., to taste)

Directions:

1. Combine sun dried tomatoes, cherry tomatoes, and arugula in a large bowl.

2. Top with vinegar, olive oil, salt, and pepper then toss to evenly coat.

3. Serve, and enjoy.

Carrot and Avocado Salad

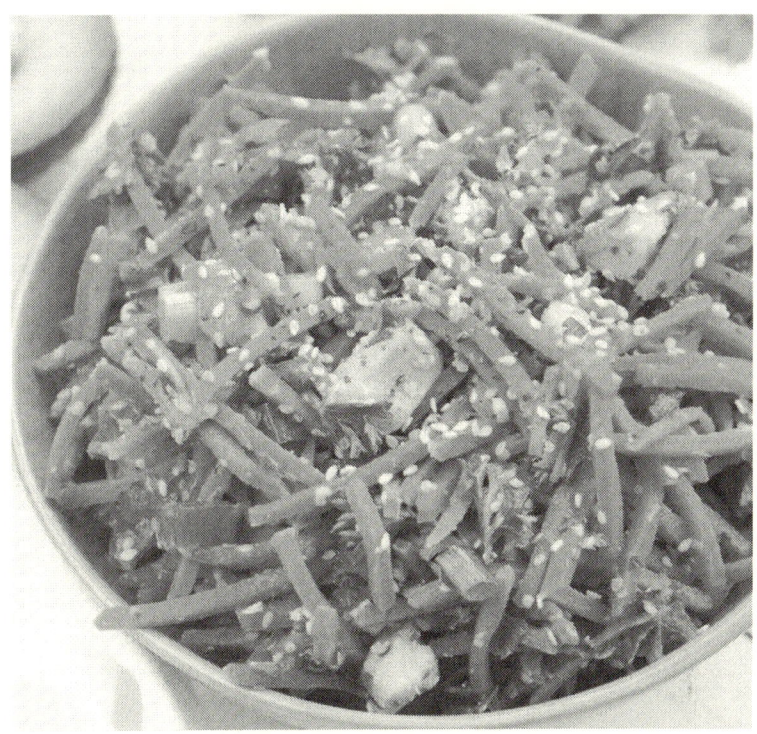

Carrots are not only great for your vision, but also carries great cancer fighting properties like Beta-carotene, folate, and a large number of vitamins.

Serving Size: 2

Overall Time: 25 Minutes

Ingredients:

- Avocado (1 large, pitted, diced)
- Carrot (4 medium, peeled, grated)
- Balsamic vinegar (1 tsp.)
- Sunflower seeds (1 tbsp., toasted)
- Salt and pepper (¼ tsp., to taste)

Directions:

1. In a medium bowl, add carrot, and avocado. Top with vinegar, salt, sunflower seeds, and pepper, then toss to evenly coat.

2. Tightly cover, and set to chill for about 20 minutes, before serving. Enjoy.

Beet, Carrot Ginger Salad

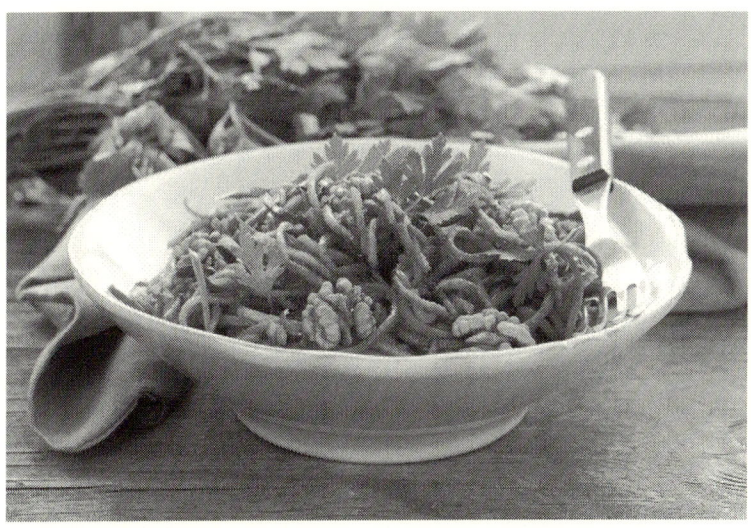

Continuing on our journey down Beta-carotene lane, we have another colorful, nutritious, delicious salad filled with fat - soluble vitamins.

Serving Size: 1

Overall Time: 15 Minutes

Ingredients:

- Beets (½ cup, peeled, grated)
- Carrots (½ cup, grated)
- Apple juice (2 tbsp.)
- Olive oil (1 tbsp., extra-virgin)
- Ginger (½ tsp., minced)
- Salt (1/8 tsp.)

Directions:

1. In a small bowl, add your carrots, and beets then, stir to combine.

2. In a separate bowl, combine all your remaining ingredients and whisk to fully incorporate.

3. Drizzle your dressing over the salad, and gently toss to evenly coat.

4. Serve.

Broccoli Salad with Apples and Cranberries

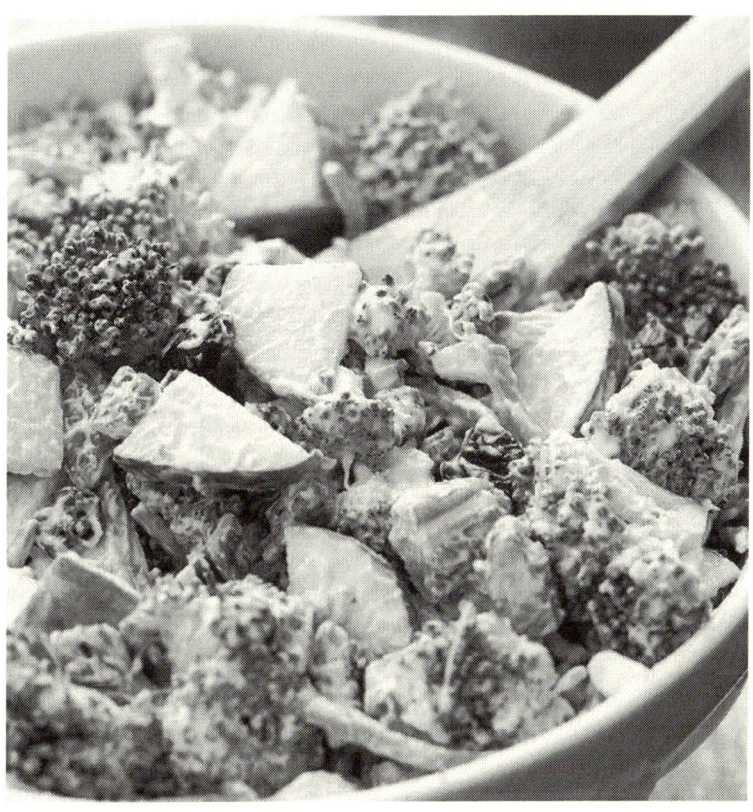

This delicious salad has a low glycemic index rating yet is so delicious, and naturally sweet that you won't want to put it down

Serving Size: 6

Overall Time: 15 Minutes

Ingredients:

- Broccoli (4 cups, cut into florets)
- Cranberries (1/2 cup, dried)
- Sunflower seeds (1/2 cup)
- Apples (3, sliced)
- Red onions (1/4 cup, chopped)
- Yogurt (1 cup, low-fat, plain)
- Dijon mustard (1 tbsp.)
- Honey (1/4 cup)

Directions:

1. In a large bowl add your onions, apples, sunflower seeds, cranberries, and broccoli, and set aside.

2. Create a dressing, by blending together honey, mustard, and yogurt in a separate bowl.

3. Drizzle your dressing over your salad, and toss to evenly coat.

4. Cover tightly, and set to chill before serving.

5. Enjoy!

Tomato, Cucumber Red Onion Salad

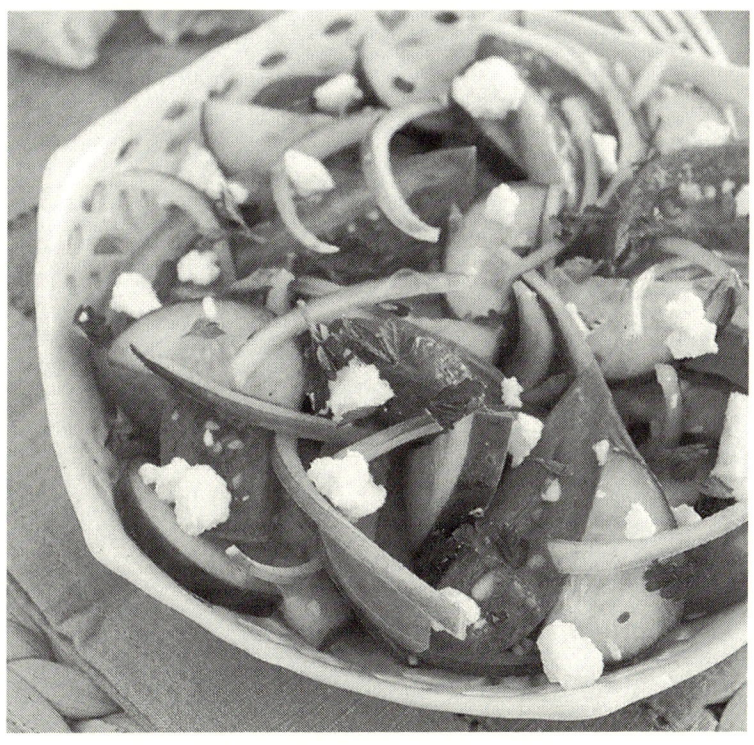

This salad has a number of anti – cancer properties is easy to prepare, tasty, easy to digest.

Serving Size: 1

Overall Time: 10 Minutes

Ingredients:

- Cucumber (2 large, washed, chopped coarsely)
- Tomato (3 large, washed, chopped coarsely)
- Red onion (2/3 cup, chopped coarsely)
- Balsamic vinegar (1/3 cup)
- White sugar (½ tbsp.)
- Olive oil (3 tbsp., extra virgin)
- Salt and pepper (1 tsp., to taste)
- Mint leaves (1 tsp., finely chopped)

Directions:

1. Add all your ingredients to a large bowl.

2. Tightly cover, hold firmly, and shake well to mix.

3. Serve, and enjoy.

ACE Salad

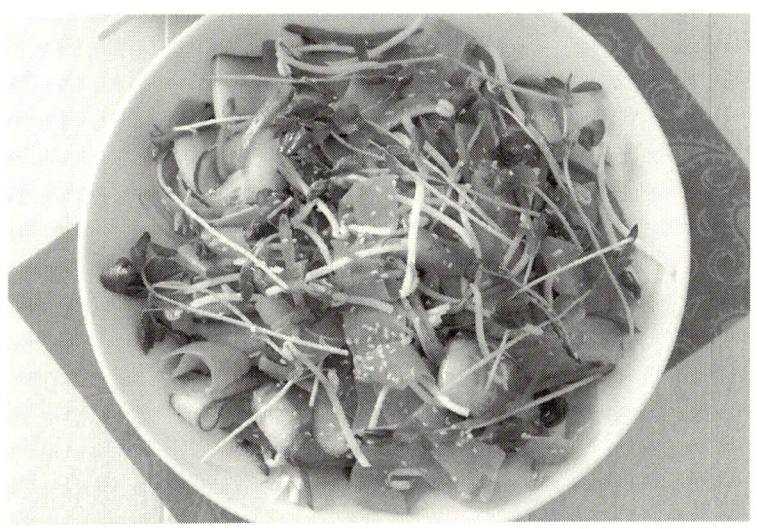

Soothe your soul with this delicious, and healthy salad that will provide you with the energy that your body.

Serving Size: 6

Overall Time: 15 Minutes

Ingredients:

- Carrots (6, sliced thinly)
- Fennel (1 bulb, sliced thinly)
- Cucumber (1, sliced thinly)
- Parsley (1 cup, chopped)
- Lemon juice (4 tbsp.)
- Olive oil (2 tbsp., extra virgin)
- Sea salt (1/4 tsp., to taste)
- Black pepper (1/4 tsp., to taste)

Directions:

1. Add your parsley, cucumber, fennel, and carrots to large bowl.

2. In a separate bowl, combine salt, pepper, oil, and lemon juice then whisk to combine.

3. Drizzle your dressing over salad. Toss gently to evenly coat, and serve.

Apple Onion Soup

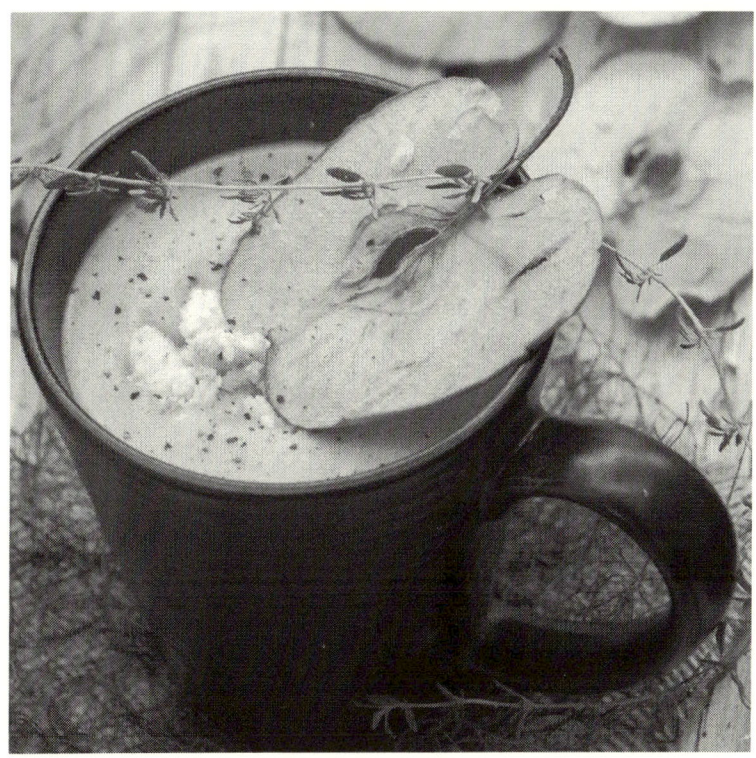

Both apples and onions have been recognized as great sources of quercetin, which greatly aids in our battle again cancer properties. This recipe uses them both to create a bowl of delicious soup.

Serving Size: 6

Overall Time: 20 Minutes

Ingredients:

- Canola oil (1 tbsp.)
- Yellow onion (2 medium, sliced)
- Leek (1 small stalk, chopped)
- Rosemary (½ tbsp., chopped)
- Thyme (½ tbsp., leaves)
- Apples (3, diced)
- Vegetable broth (6 cups, low sodium, fat-free)

Directions:

1. Set a medium saucepan with oil over medium heat, and allow to get hot.

2. Once hot, add onions and cook, while stirring, until lightly golden.

3. Add broth and allow to come to a boil.

4. Add your remaining ingredients, reduce heat to low, and let simmer for about 10 minutes.

5. Serve, and enjoy.

Tangy Tomato Basil Soup

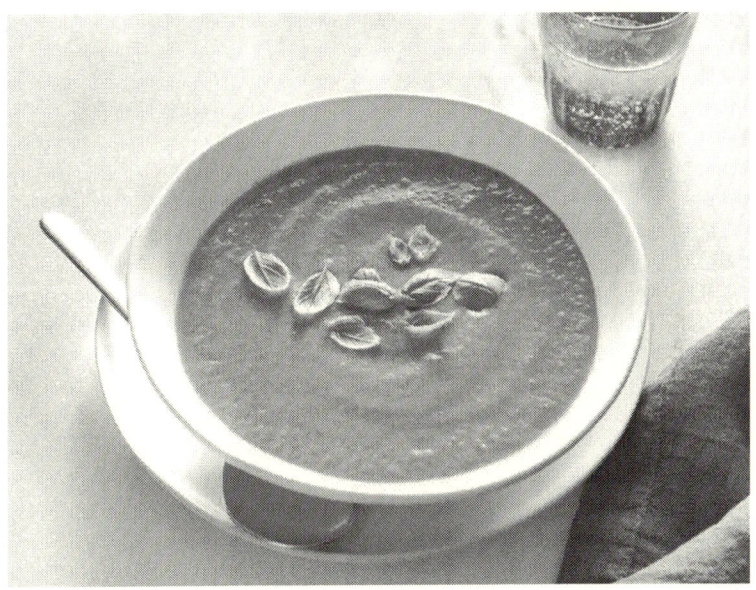

Believe it or not, a simple bowl of tomato soup provides your body with a wide range of antioxidants to help battle against cancer cells.

Serving Size: 2

Overall Time: 11 Minutes

Ingredients:

- Garlic (3 cloves, peeled, crushed)
- Shallots (3 oz., peeled, sliced)
- Olive oil (1 tbsp.)
- Stewed tomatoes (14½ oz., canned, undrained)
- Chicken broth (1½ cups)
- Apple cider vinegar (½ tsp.)
- Salt (¼ tsp.)
- Black pepper (¼ tsp.)
- Basil (2 tbsp., chopped)

Directions:

1. Add your vinegar, chicken broth, tomatoes, shallots to a food processor, and process until smooth then set aside.

2. Set a large saucepan with oil, over medium heat, and allow to get hot.

3. Once hot, add garlic then cook, while stirring, for about 30 seconds.

4. Add tomato, and chicken broth mixture, and allow to come to a boil.

5. Remove from heat, add basil, stir, and serve.

Grandma's Chicken Soup

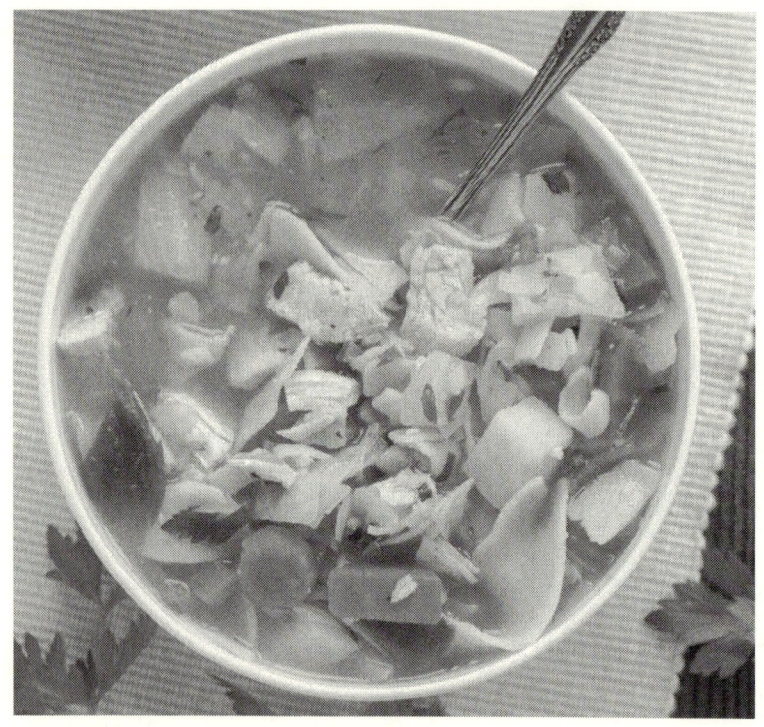

Not beats a large bowl of chicken soup, whether you are combatting a cold, or cancer.

Serving Size: 6

Overall Time: 14 Minutes

Ingredients:

- Chicken broth (4 cups, low-sodium, fat – free)
- Onion (1, chopped)
- Sweet potato (3/4 cup, diced)
- Turnip (3/4 cup, diced)
- Celery (2 ribs, diced)
- Carrot (2, sliced)
- Parsley (½ cup, chopped)
- Chicken (2 cups, cooked, diced)

Directions:

1. Set a large saucepan with your broth over medium heat, and allow to come to a boil.

2. Add vegetables, stir, and reduce the heat to low, and allow to simmer covered until your vegetables become for tender.

3. Add chicken, stir, and leave to simmer for another 4 minutes.

4. Serve, and enjoy.

Beet and Carrot Soup

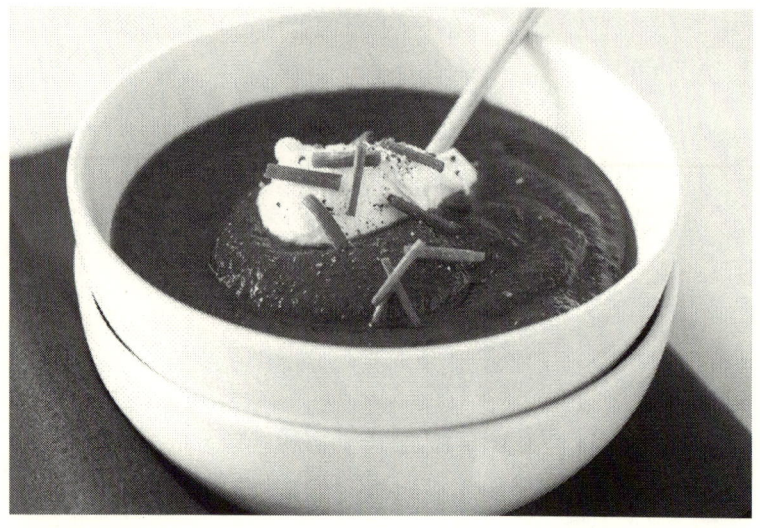

This delicious bowl of crimson soup is nutrient dense, and delicious.

Serving Size: 4

Overall Time: 40 Minutes

Ingredients:

- Beets (3 medium, peeled, diced)
- Olive oil (1 tbsp.)
- Onion (1 cup, chopped)
- Carrot (1 lb., diced)
- Ginger (1 tbsp., minced)
- Garlic (1 clove, minced)
- Vegetable stock (6 cups)

Directions:

1. Set a large saucepan with oil over medium heat, and allow to get hot.

2. Add onion, and cook, while stirring, until golden brown.

3. Add garlic, and ginger then continue to cook, while stirring, for 2 minutes.

4. Add stock, carrots, and beets. Stir, and reduce the heat to low.

5. Allow to simmer, while covered, until carrots, and beets become fork tender (about 25 minutes).

6. Transfer your soup, in batches to a food processor, and purée until smooth.

7. Season to taste with salt, and pepper then serve.

Broccoli and Barley Soup

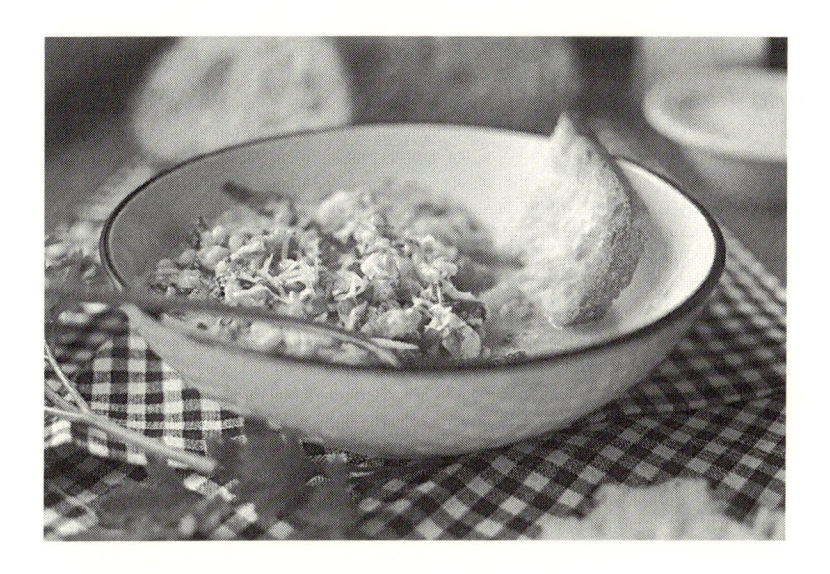

This nutritious soup provides a delicious bowl of sulforaphane, which is an interesting compound that aids in the prevention, and possible reduction of lung cancer tumors.

Serving Size: 6

Overall Time: 22 Minutes

Ingredients:

- Yellow onion (¼ cup, chopped)
- Carrot (1, peeled, diced)
- Celery (1 rib, chopped finely)
- Olive oil (1 tbsp., extra virgin)
- Broccoli (4 cups, cut into florets)
- Barley (½ cup, pearled, cooked)
- Vegetable broth (5 cups)
- Stewed tomatoes (14½ oz.)
- Garlic (4 cloves, minced)
- Marjoram (¼ tsp., dried)
- Thyme leaves (1 tsp.)
- Salt and pepper (¼ tsp., to taste)

Directions:

1. Set a stock pot with oil, over medium heat, and allow to get oil.

2. Add onions, celery, and carrots and cook, while stirring, until fork tender (about 5 minutes)

3. Add broth and allow to come to a boil.

4. Once boiling, reduce the heat to low, and add broccoli. Allow to simmer, covered, until broccoli becomes fork tender.

5. Add remaining ingredients, and continue simmering for another 2 minutes.

6. Season to taste with salt and pepper.

7. Serve, and enjoy.

Scandinavian Blueberry Soup

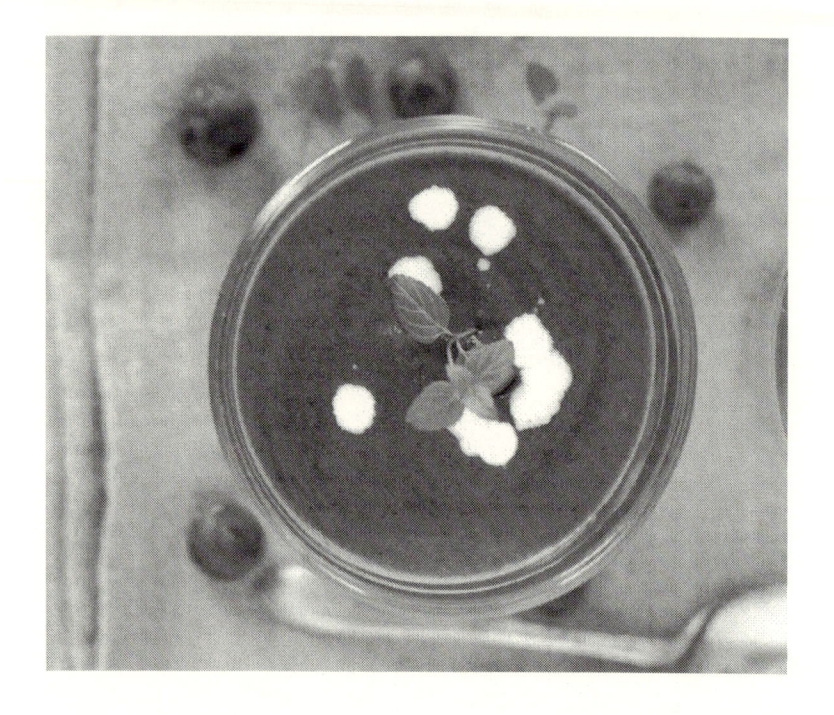

This tasty soup is popular in Scandinavia. It allows you to enjoy all the nutritional properties of blueberries with a natural sweetness that even the kids can appreciate.

Serving Size: 3

Overall Time: 20 Minutes

Ingredients:

- Blueberries (4 cups)
- Water (2 cups)
- Sugar (1/2 cup)
- Potato starch (4 tbsp)

Directions:

1. Set a large saucepan over medium heat with your water, sugar, and blueberries then allow to come to a boil.

2. Create a smooth paste, by mixing your potato starch, and a few drops of water together in a small bowl. Stir into the saucepan, and reduce the heat to low, and leave to cook until the soup thickens.

3. Serve, and enjoy.

Green Tea Mango Blast

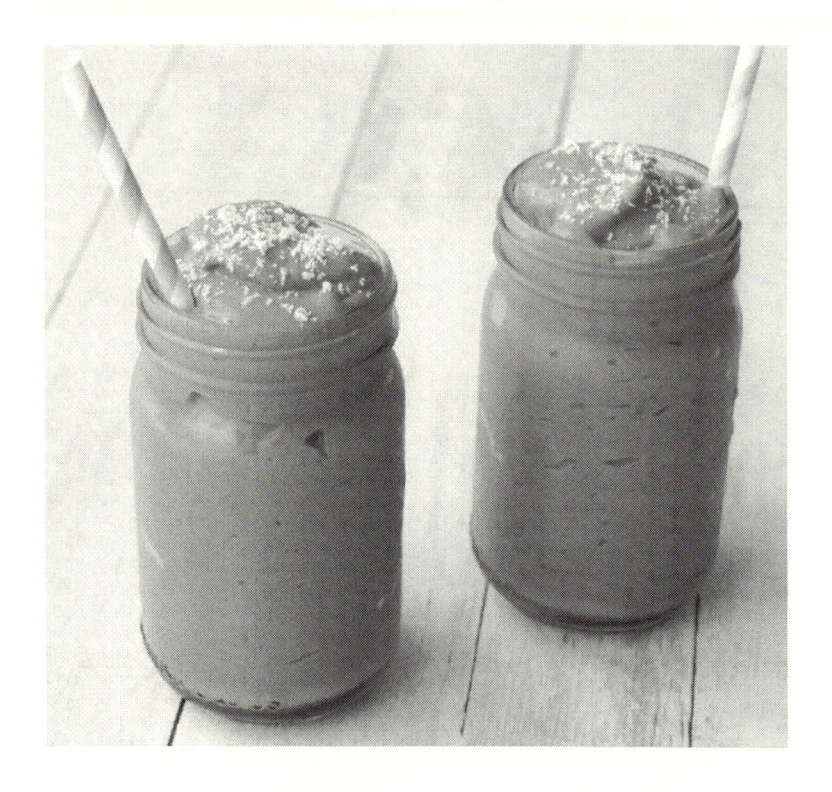

This refreshing smoothie is the perfect afternoon drink to allow you to get your anti – cancer antioxidant compounds.

Serving Size: 2

Overall Time: 5 Minutes

Ingredients:

- Mango (2 cups, peeled, chopped)
- Green tea (1 cup)
- Honey (1 tbsp.)
- Ginger (½ inch, peeled, chopped finely)
- Ice (1 cup, crushed)

Directions:

1. Add all your ingredients to a blender, and process until smooth.

2. Serve, and enjoy!

Catechin-Rich Ice Tea

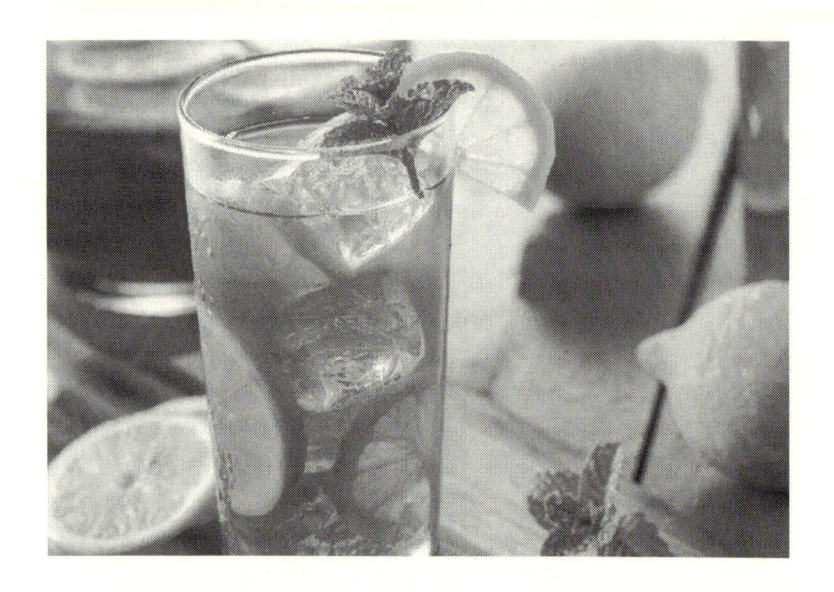

If you are an iced tea lover, this recipe allows you to enjoy a refreshing glass filled with catechins that have been proven to provide a large number of anti-cancer properties.

Serving Size: 2

Overall Time: 6 Minutes

Ingredients:

- Water (2 cups)
- Green tea leaves (2½ tsp., loose)
- Lemon juice (3 tbsp.)

Directions:

1. Set a small sauce pan with water over high heat, then allow to come to a boil.

2. Add green tea leaves, cover, and remove from heat. Allow to steep for about 5 minutes.

3. Strain tea through a fine mesh strainer.

4. Add lemon juice, stir, and set in the refrigerator to chill before serving. Enjoy!

Raspberry Blueberry Smoothie

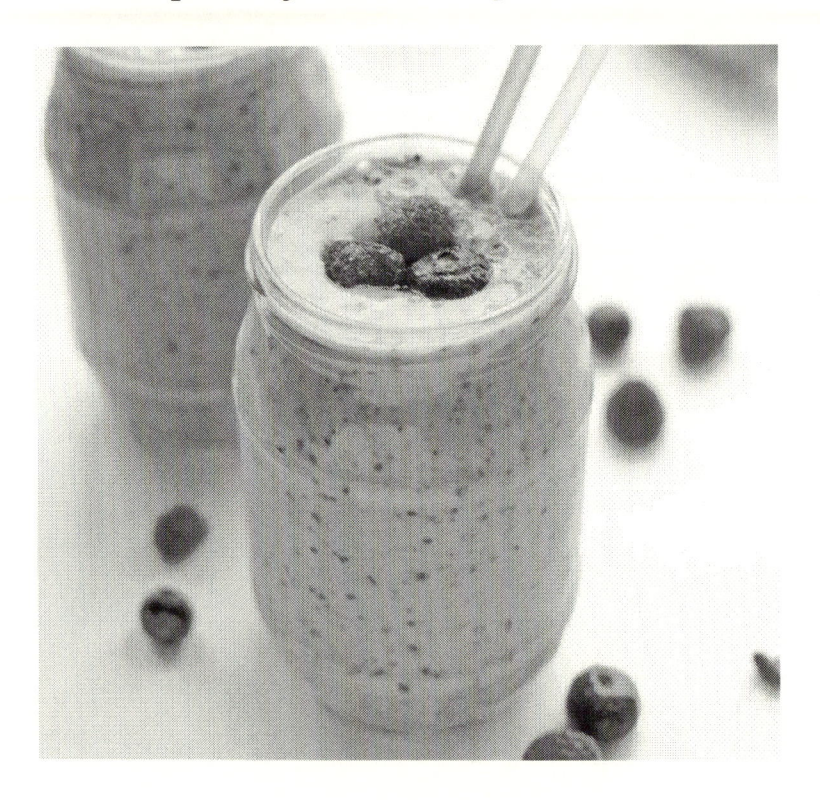

This delicious smoothie is made using two popular cancer fighting fruits: raspberries and blueberries. Above all, it is delicious, and perfect for a warm day.

Serving Size: 3

Overall Time: 5 Minutes

Ingredients:

- Raspberries (1 cup, fresh)
- Blueberries (1 cup, wild)
- Rice milk (3/4 cup)
- Ice (3/4 cup, crushed)
- Flaxseed (1 tbsp., ground)

Directions:

1. Add all your ingredients to a blender then allow to process until smooth.

2. Serve, and enjoy!

Blueberry Pecan Antioxidant Muffins

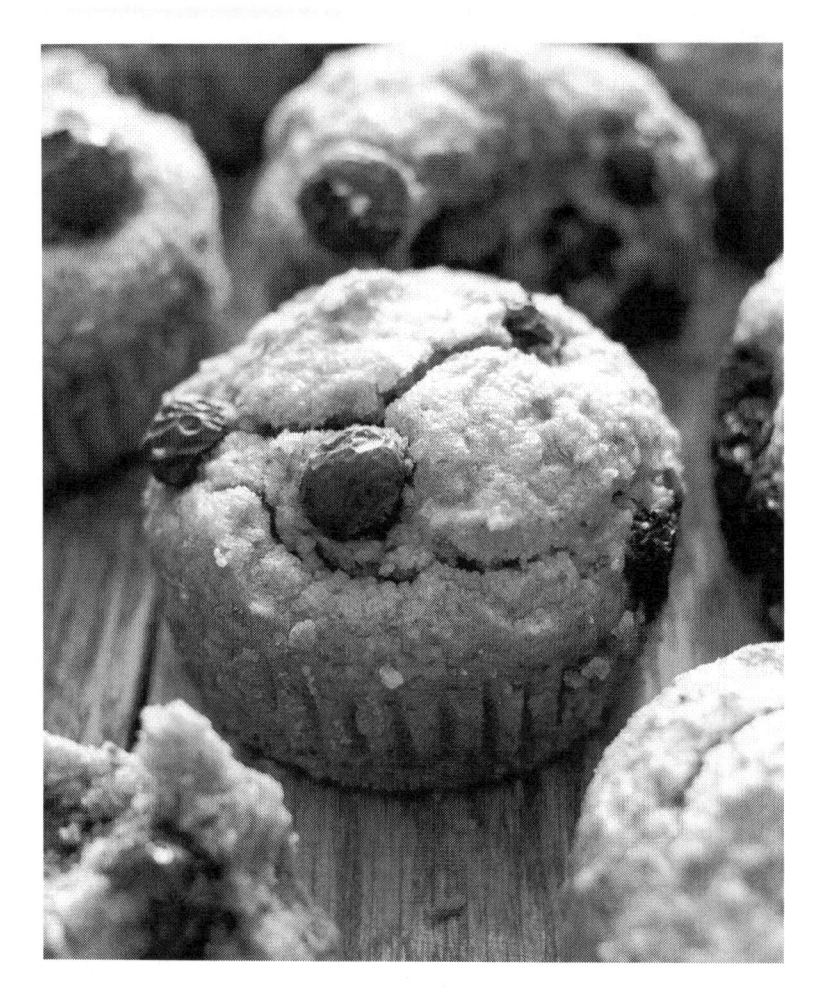

These delicious muffins are made from two powerhouses when it comes to antioxidants that make them great dessert options for cancer patients.

Serving Size: 6-8

Overall Time: 50 Minutes

Ingredients:

- Flour (1 cup, whole wheat)
- Brown sugar (1/3 cup)
- Baking powder (1/2 tsp.)
- Pecans (1/3 cup, chopped)
- Salt (1/4 tsp.)
- Blueberries (1 cup)
- Almond Milk (1/4 cup)
- Egg (1 large)

Directions:

1. Set your oven to preheat to 350 degrees F.

2. Add salt, pecans, baking powder, sugar, and flour in a large bowl.

3. Add all your wet ingredients to a separate bowl then whisk to combine.

4. Slowly add your wet ingredients to the dry bowl, and stir to combine.

5. Transfer the batter evenly into a lined muffin tin.

6. Set to bake until done (about 30 minutes).

7. Lightly cool, then serve.

Low-Fat Apple and Raspberry Crumble

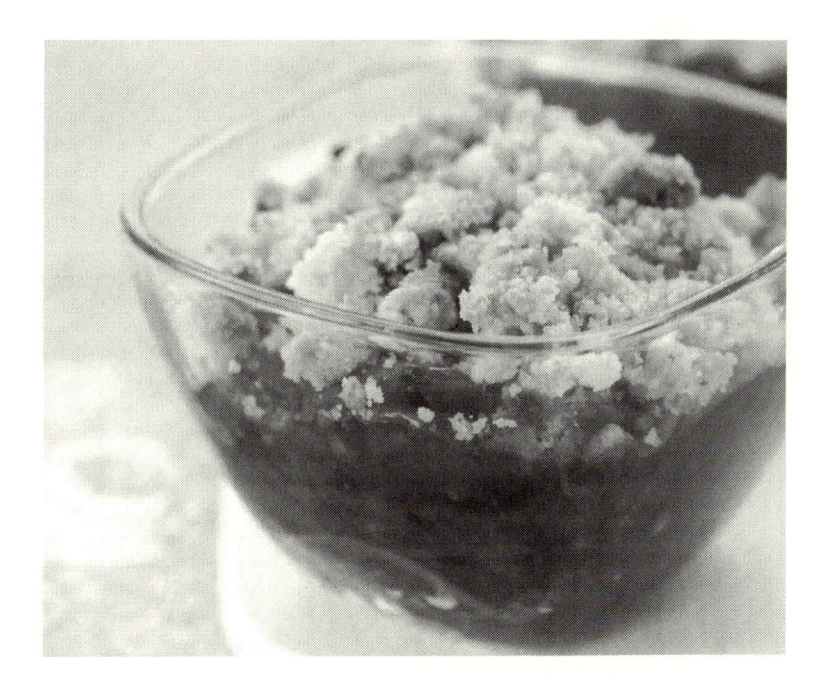

Here is a healthy, low – fat dessert that will kick your taste buds back into high gear.

Serving Size: 6

Overall Time: 55 Minutes

Ingredients:

- Apples (5 large, Granny Smith, sliced finely)
- Raspberries (1 cup)
- Apple juice (2 cups)
- Oats (2 cups, rolled)
- Butter (2 tbsp.)
- Brown sugar (2 tbsp)
- Cinnamon (2 tsp., ground)
- Cloves (1/2 tsp.)

Directions:

1. Set your oven to preheat to 350 degrees F.

2. Layer raspberries, and apple in a lightly greased baking dish, then top with apple juice.

3. Add spices, sugar, and oats in a medium bowl. Add butter and evenly disperse by massaging with fingers.

4. Transfer evenly to your baking dish over the apples, and raspberries.

5. Set to bake until crisp, and golden brown (about 45 - 60 minutes).

6. Serve, or chill.

Buckwheat Crepes with Prune Compote

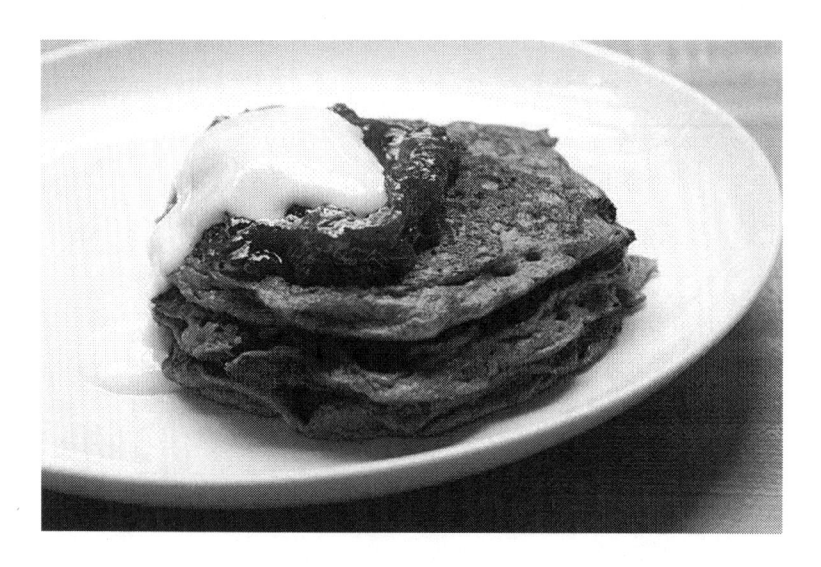

This delicious dessert provides your body with the rutin compound, to help fight off cancer cells.

Serving Size: 8

Overall Time: 30 Minutes

Ingredients:

- Eggs (2, large, beaten)
- Rice milk (1¼ cups)
- Buckwheat flour (2/3 cup)
- Quinoa flour (1/3 cup)
- Canola Oil (1 tbsp.)
- Salt (1/2 tsp.)
- Prunes (8 oz., pitted, softened in warm water)
- Water (1 cup)
- Brown sugar (1 tbsp.)
- Apple Juice (1 tbsp.)
- Vegetable cooking spray (1 can)

Directions:

1. Add eggs, salt, oil, quinoa flour, buckwheat flour, and rice milk in a medium bowl then whisk well to combine.

2. Set a large skillet over medium heat. Lightly grease with cooking spray.

3. Add 1/3 cup of your batter to the hot skillet in the center. Quickly rotate the skillet to allow your batter to run covering the entire bottom of the pan.

4. All crepe to cook until the top becomes slightly bubbly (about 2 minutes). Flip crepe and continue cooking for another minute.

5. Transfer from hot skillet, and set aside. Repeat steps 2 – 5 until all the batter has been cooked.

6. Set a medium saucepan over medium heat with apple juice, sugar, water, and prunes.

7. Allow to come to a boil then reduce heat to low. Continue to simmer until prunes become tender (about 15 minutes).

8. Slightly cool prune compote, and serve on top of crepes.

Flourless Chocolate Cake

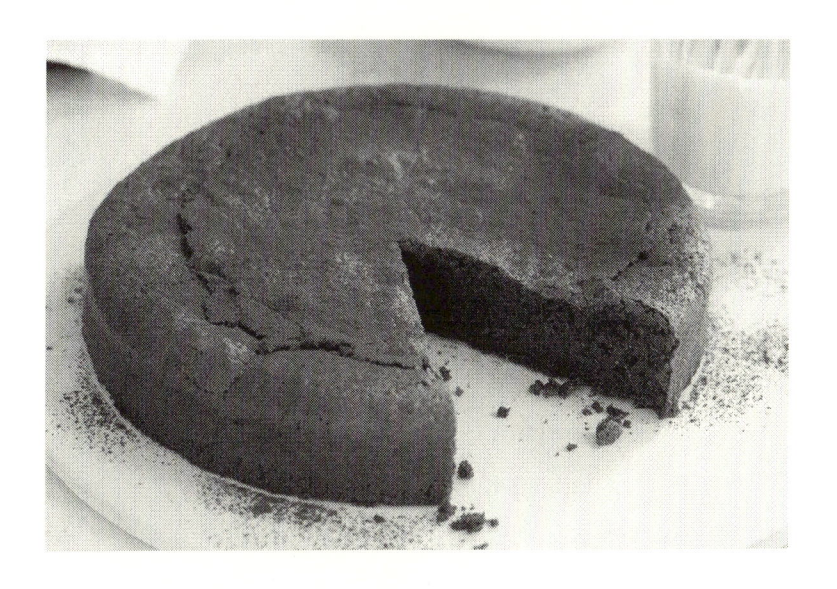

This delicious chocolate cake is made from black beans! It is low in calories, delicious, and nutritious.

Serving Size: 9

Overall Time: 55 Minutes

Ingredients:

- Black bean (1½ cups, cooked)
- Eggs (4, large)
- Mint extract (1 tbsp.)
- Stevia (1 tsp.)
- Vegetable oil (5 tbsp.)
- Honey (1/3 cup)
- Cocoa powder (6 tbsp., dark, unsweetened)
- Baking powder (1 tsp.)
- Baking soda (1/2 tsp.)
- Salt (a pinch)
- Mint Leaves (a few for garnish)

Directions:

1. Set oven to preheat to 350 degrees F.

2. Add mint, honey, oil, stevia, beans and 2 eggs to blender then process until smooth. Set aside.

3. Add baking powder, baking soda, and cocoa powder to a small bowl.

4. In a large bowl, whisk together your 2 remaining eggs.

5. Add your bean batter and mix to combine.

6. Add cocoa powder mixture and stir vigorously until fully combined.

7. Transfer batter to a lightly greased cake pan (preferably 9-inch).

8. Set to bake until cooked (about 35 - 45 minutes).

9. Cool, top with your favorite frosting, and enjoy.

Rice Pudding with Blueberry Sauce

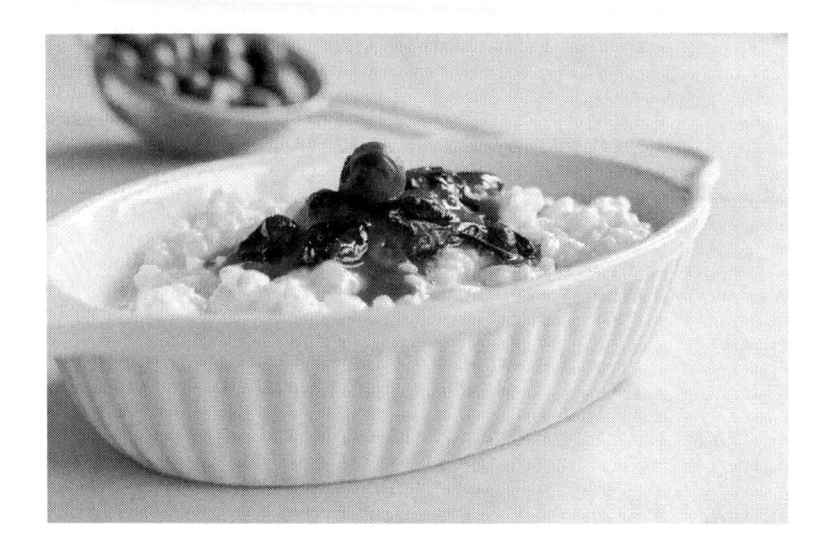

Spin your brown rice into this delicious cup of rice pudding.

Serving Size: 8

Overall Time: 1 Hour 26 Minutes

Ingredients:

- Brown basmati rice (1 cup)
- Water (2 cups)
- Salt (1/2 tsp.)
- Rice milk (3 cups)
- Brown sugar (1/3 cup)
- Cinnamon (1/2 tsp., ground)
- Potato starch (1 tbsp.)
- Blueberry Sauce
- Blueberries (2 cups, crushed)
- Sugar (1/3 cup)
- Water (1 tbsp.)

Directions:

1. Set a medium saucepan over high heat with salt, water, and rice. Allow to come to a boil and then reduce the heat to low.

2. Continue simmering, covered, until the water has been fully absorbed (about 40 minutes).

3. Add remaining pudding ingredients, except potato starch, and continue to cook for another 10 minutes, stirring occasionally.

4. Add potato starch, and enough water to just cover it in a small bowl. Stir to create a smooth paste, then add into the rice mixture.

5. Continue to cook, while stirring, until the mixture thickens into a pudding (about 6 minutes).

6. Transfer the mixture to a bowl. Tightly cover, and set to chill for about 2 hours in the refrigerator.

7. While chilling, add water, sugar, and blueberries to a small pot, over medium heat.

8. Allow to come to a boil and reduce heat to low, and simmer for about 1 minute.

9. Serve blueberry sauce on top of your rice pudding.

10. Enjoy.

Barley Soup with Beans and Basil

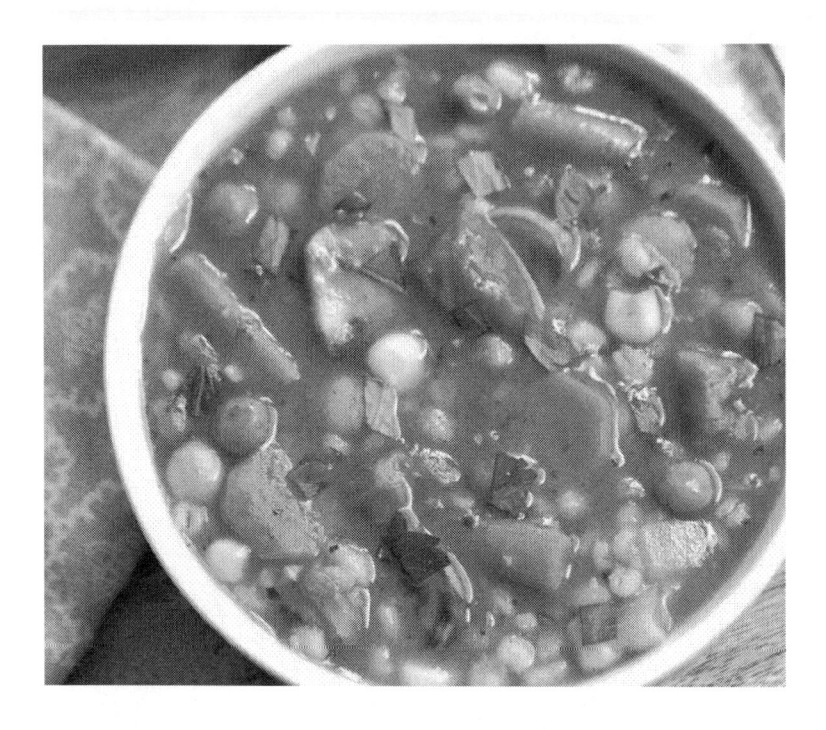

Get half your daily dose of selenium, with this filling, and tasty bowl of soup.

Serving Size: 6

Overall Time: 20 Minutes

Ingredients:

- Yellow onion (1/4 cup, chopped)
- Carrot (1, peeled, diced)
- Celery (1 rib, chopped finely)
- Olive oil (1 tbsp., extra virgin)
- Vegetable broth (5 cups)
- Barley (1/2 cup, pearled, cooked)
- White beans (1/2 cup, cooked)
- Tomatoes (1/4 cup, canned)
- Garlic (4 cloves, minced)
- Basil (3 tbsp, chopped)
- Rosemary (1/2 tsp., dried)
- Salt and pepper (1/4 tsp., to taste)

Directions:

1. Set a large saucepan with oil over medium heat, and allow to get hot.

2. Once hot, add onion, carrots, and celery and cook, while stirring, until soft (about 3 minutes).

3. Add broth, and allow to come to a boil.

4. Add remaining ingredients, stir, and reduce to low heat. Allow soup to simmer for another 2 minutes.

5. Season to taste, and serve.

Nourishing Nettle Soup

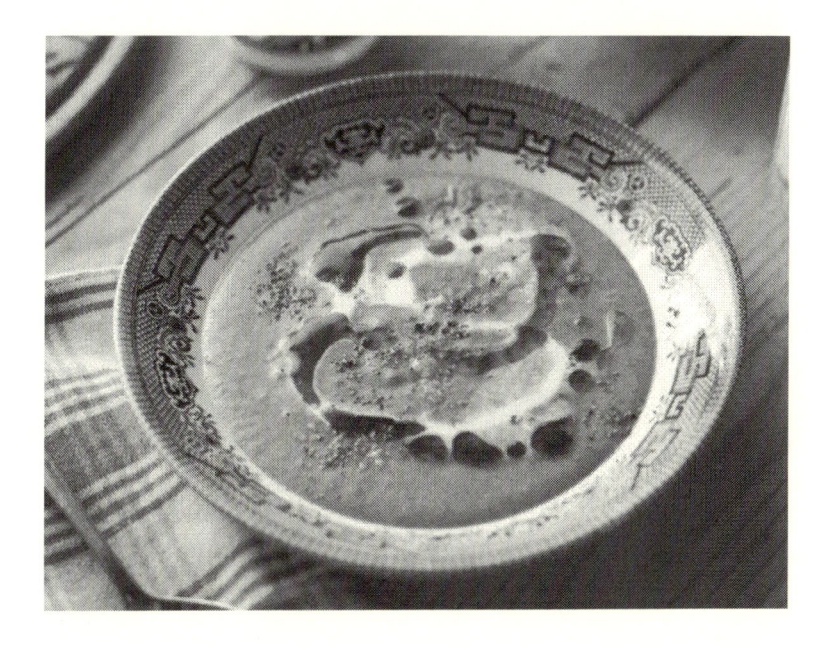

If you have never had nettle before, you need to try it in this soup. This soup is not only delicious but also packed a variety of vitamins and other antioxidants.

Serving Size: 4

Overall Time: 25 Minutes

Ingredients:

- Nettle tips (6 oz., young)
- Spinach (4 oz., washed, chopped coarsely)
- Olive oil (2 tbsp.)
- Shallots (2, chopped)
- Water (2 cups)
- Milk (2 cups, skimmed)
- Flour (3 tbsp.)
- White pepper (1/4 tsp.)
- Nutmeg (1/8 tsp.)
- Salt (1 tsp., to taste)

Directions:

1. Set a large saucepan with oil over medium heat and allow to get hot.

2. Once hot, add onion and cook, while stirring, until golden brown.

3. Add spinach, nettle, and water, and allow to come to a boil. Allow to cook until greens become tender.

4. Transfer to a blender, and puree until smooth then return to saucepan over medium heat.

5. In a small bowl, combine your flour, and milk then stir until a smooth paste is formed. Stir the mixture into your soup.

6. Allow the soup to return to a boil, reduce the heat, and let simmer until soup thickens.

7. Add nutmeg, then season to taste with pepper and salt.

8. Serve, and enjoy.

Cold Minty Watercress Soup

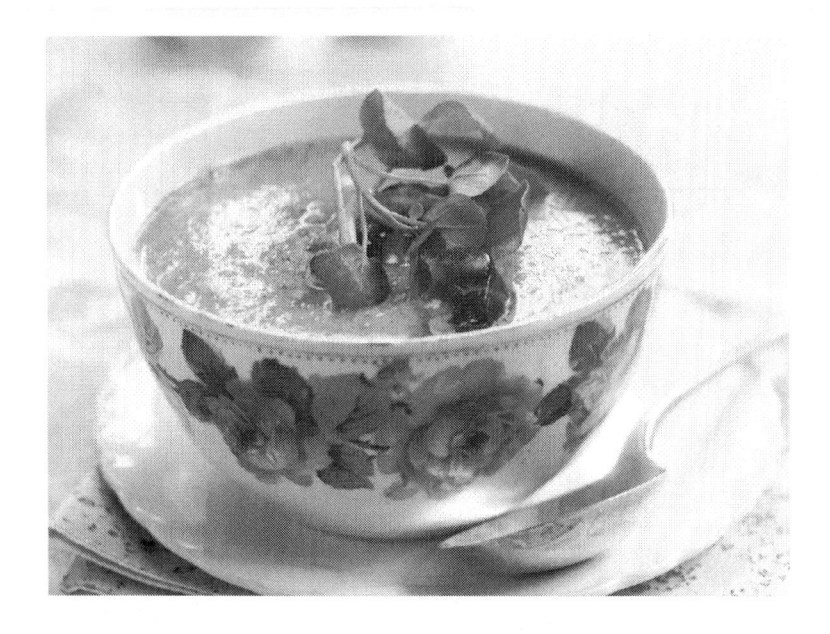

Enjoy the nutritional benefits of watercress, and mint in this deliciously refreshing bowl of soup.

Serving Size: 4

Overall Time: 15 Minutes

Ingredients:

- Cucumbers (4, large, peeled, diced)
- Watercress (1 cup)
- Apple cider vinegar (2 tbsp.)
- Olive oil (1 tbsp., extra-virgin)
- Mint (3/4 cup, leaves)
- Oregano (2 tbsp.)
- Chives (3 tbsp., chopped)
- Yogurt (1½ cups, plain)
- Salt and pepper (1 tsp. each, to taste)

Directions:

1. Add your chives, cucumbers, oregano, mint, oil, vinegar, and watercress to a food processor, and puree until smooth.

2. Season to taste with salt and pepper, add yogurt, stir, then transfer to a bowl.

3. Cover tightly, and set to refrigerate for about 2 hours before serving. Enjoy!

Whole-wheat Pasta with Nettle Pesto

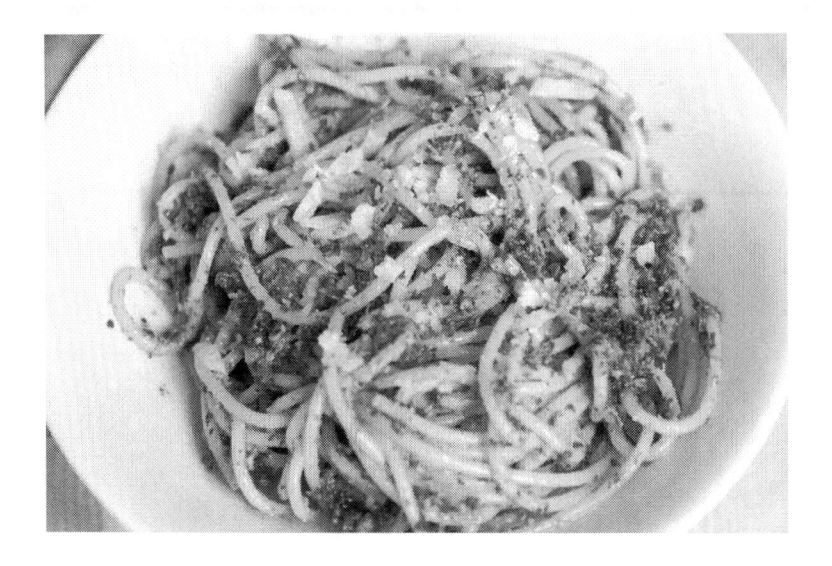

Tantalize your taste buds with this interesting plate of pasta.

Serving Size: 4

Overall Time: 17 Minutes

Ingredients:

- Nettle leaves (2 cups, young, blanched)
- Garlic (4 cloves, peeled)
- Walnut (1/3 cup, chopped)
- Parmesan cheese (1/3 cup, grated)
- Olive oil (1/3 cup, extra-virgin)
- Pasta (12 oz., whole-wheat)

Directions:

1. Set your pasta to cook using the directions on the package.

2. While that cooks, add walnuts, garlic, olive oil and nettle leaves to your food processor. Process until a smooth sauce is created. Add grated parmesan cheese, stir and set aside.

3. Drain water from pasta when done, add nettle pesto and stir to evenly coat.

4. Serve, and enjoy.

Shrimp and Mushroom Risotto

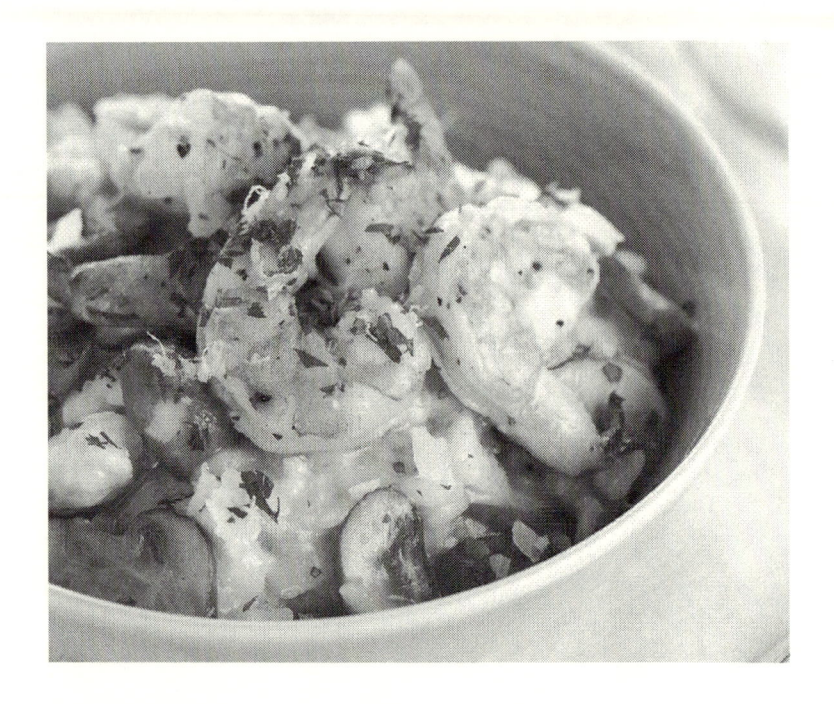

This risotto is easy to make, delicious, and nutritious.

Serving Size: 3

Overall Time: 35 Minutes

Ingredients:

- Olive oil (3 tbsp.)
- Crimini mushrooms (1/4 lb., cleaned, stemmed, diced)
- Shrimp (1/4 lb., peeled, deveined)
- Garlic (1 clove, minced)
- Onion (1, chopped finely)
- Brown rice (1 2/3 cups)
- Vegetable broth (4 1/4 cups)
- Chives (3 tbsp., chopped)
- Frozen peas (1/4 lb., thawed)
- Salt and pepper (1 tsp., to taste)

Directions:

1. Set a large saucepan with 2 tbsp. oil over medium heat to get how.

2. Add shrimp and mushrooms then season to taste.

3. Allow to cook, while stirring, until shrimp is cooked through (about 5 minutes). Set aside.

4. Heat the rest of your oil into the saucepan. Add onion, and garlic, and sauté for until soft.

5. Add rice and allow to toast slightly in the pot pan. Begin pouring in half of your broth and cook while stirring until almost fully absorbed.

6. Once absorbed add in a bit more broth, and continue to cook while stirring. Continue adding in your broth a little at a time until almost rice is almost cooked.

7. Add remaining ingredients, stir, and allow to continue cooking, while stirring for a few more minutes. Serve, and enjoy.

Original Bircher Muesli

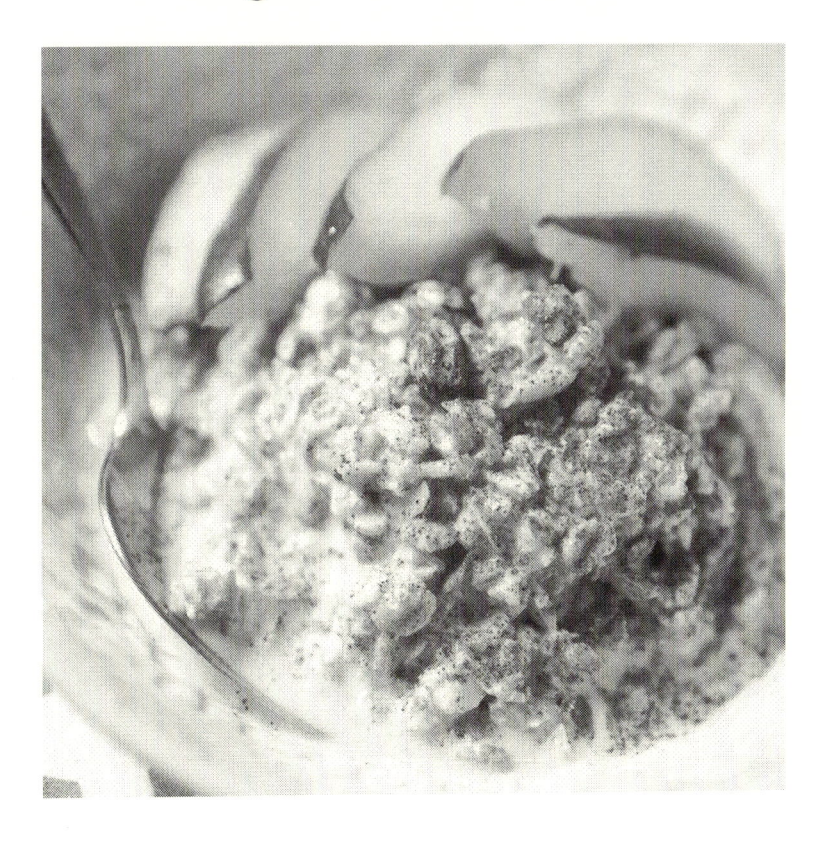

This delicious Muesli is deliciously sweet.

Serving Size: 1

Overall Time: 15 Minutes

Ingredients:

- Oats (1 tbsp., rolled)
- Water (3 tbsp.)
- Milk (1 tbsp., sweetened condensed)
- Lemon juice (2 tsp.)
- Apples (2, grated)
- Hazelnuts (1 tbsp., chopped)

Directions:

1. Add water and oats to a medium bowl, stir, and set to soak overnight in the refrigerator.

2. Add lemon juice, condensed milk, and apples then stir well to combine.

3. Top with hazelnuts, and serve.

Oat and Wheat Germ Muesli with Apples

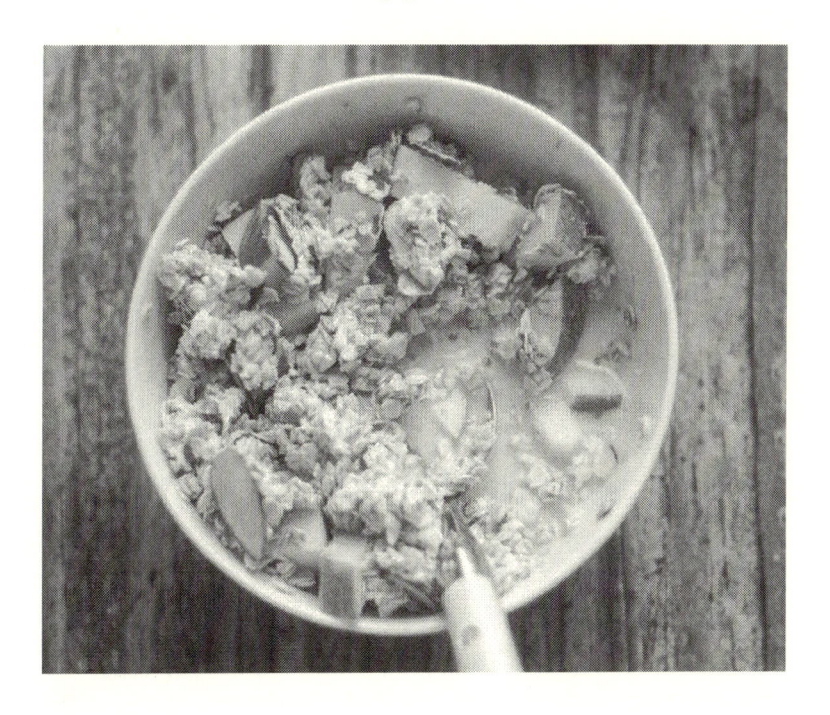

Enjoy this delicious bowl of Muesli, and get a serving of zinc, selenium, and vitamin E from each bite.

Serving Size: 4

Overall Time: 15 Minutes

Ingredients:

- Oats (1½ cups, toasted)
- Wheat germ (1/2 cup)
- Cinnamon (2 tsp., ground)
- Apples (1½ cups, diced)
- Brown sugar (2 tbsp.)

Directions:

1. Set your oven to preheat to 325 degrees F.

2. Add cinnamon, sugar, and oats in a medium bowl.

3. Stir to combine, and transfer evenly to a lined baking tray.

4. Set to toast, stirring occasionally (about 10 minutes).

5. Cool slightly, then transfer to a large bowl. Add wheat germ, and stir.

6. Top with apples, and serve.

Conclusion

We are elated that you were able to complete all 30 delicious life altering recipes to combat lung cancer. The next step from here is to continue practicing until you have perfected each one. After that, you can always find another amazing journey to partake in from cuisines across the globe in another one of our books. We hope to see you again soon. Happy cooking!

Author's Afterthoughts

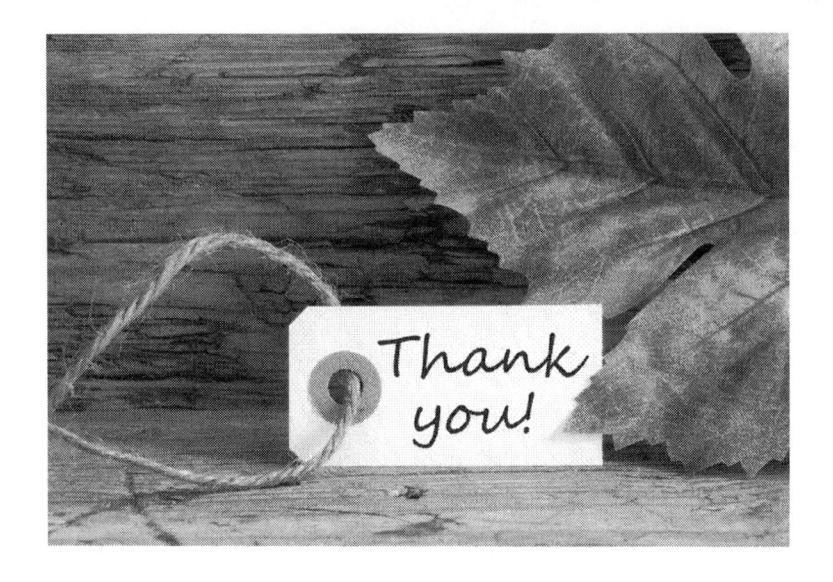

Thanks ever so much to each of my cherished readers for investing the time to read this book!

I know you could have picked from many other books but you chose this one. So a big thanks for downloading this book and reading all the way to the end.

If you enjoyed this book or received value from it, I'd like to ask you for a favor. Please take a few minutes to post an honest and heartfelt review on Amazon.com. Your support does make a difference and helps to benefit other people.

Thanks!

Daniel Humphreys

About the Author

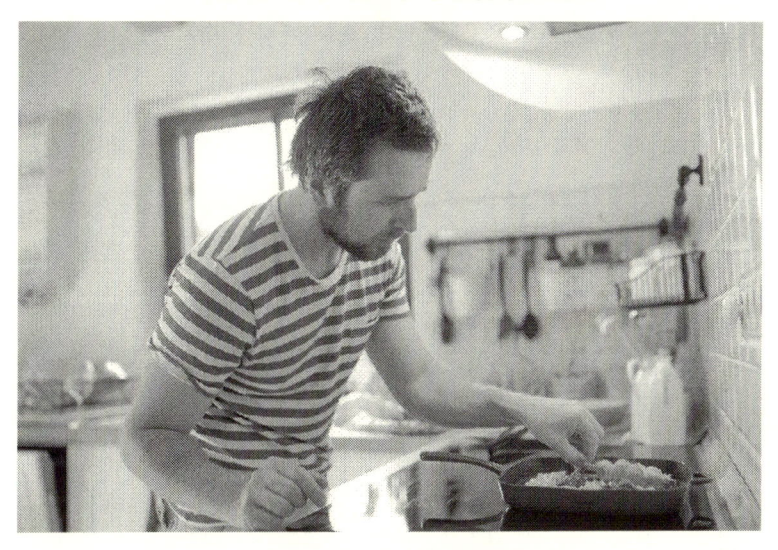

Daniel Humphreys

Many people will ask me if I am German or Norman, and my answer is that I am 100% unique! Joking aside, I owe my cooking influence mainly to my mother who was British! I can certainly make a mean Sheppard's pie, but when it comes to preparing Bratwurst sausages and drinking beer with friends, I am also all in!

I am taking you on this culinary journey with me and hope you can appreciate my diversified background. In my 15 years career as a chef, I never had a dish returned to me by one of clients, so that should say something about me! Actually, I will take that back. My worst critic is my four years old son, who refuses to taste anything that is green color. That shall pass, I am sure.

My hope is to help my children discover the joy of cooking and sharing their creations with their loved ones, like I did all my life. When you develop a passion for cooking and my suspicious is that you have one as well, it usually sticks for life. The best advice I can give anyone as a professional chef is invest. Invest your time, your heart in each meal you are creating. Invest also a little money in good cooking hardware and quality ingredients. But most of all enjoy every meal you prepare with YOUR friends and family!

Made in the USA
Middletown, DE
13 January 2022